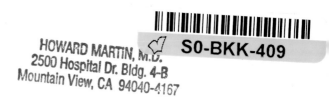

S0-BKK-409

stop the
HEARTBURN

*What you can do to reduce
your symptoms of one of
America's most common
health problems.*

© 1996 David S. Utley, M.D.

Library of Congress Catalog Card Number 96-5675
ISBN: 0-9650928-0-1
Printed in the United States

Published by:

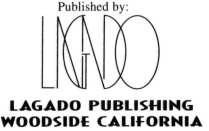

**LAGADO PUBLISHING
WOODSIDE CALIFORNIA**

Burning Fact

One hundred million people in the United
States experience heartburn and other
reflux symptoms monthly. Most of these
individuals can eliminate these symptoms
without relying on medications.

■ ■ ■

what others are *SAYING* about
STOP THE HEARTBURN

Millions of Americans suffer from gastroesophageal reflux disease, and many do not even know what they have! In this book, Dr. Utley has provided both the patient and the physician with excellent information which should help in the diagnosis and treatment of this disease. An excellent addition to both the patient and physician library.

> *Kenneth H. Cooper, M.D., M.P.H.*
> *Author of "Aerobics" and many other health titles*
> *Chairman, Cooper Clinic, Dallas*

This is a paperback guide to relief for heartburn, indigestion, difficulty swallowing, sour taste and hoarseness, written by a Stanford University Hospital otolaryngologist. Utley notes that while Americans devour medications for heartburn and related problems, lifestyle changes can also help and should be tried first. The book is neatly organized and full of practical recommendations.

> *The Los Angeles Times*
> *Health Section*
> *February 21, 1996*

Gastroesophageal reflux disease (GERD) is a common malady that can be controlled in many cases by simple methods without expensive medications. *Stop the Heartburn* discusses the causes of GERD in a very readable manner and provides a graded approach to treatment that makes good sense. I highly recommend it.

> *Richard L. Goode, M.D.*
> *Past President*
> *American Academy of Otolaryngology/Head and Neck Surgery*

Almost all of the pregnant women in my practice complain of heartburn and reflux symptoms. Anti-heartburn medications generally are not an option for these women, so we recommend the information found in *Stop the Heartburn* to reduce their symptoms. It's a great book and I highly recommend it.

> *Susan M. Hinrichs, M.D.*
> *Obstetrics and Gynecology*
> *Palo Alto, California*

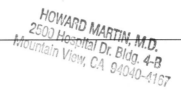

In an effort to reduce medical costs, health care is moving increasingly towards prevention and wellness. In this environment, Stop the Heartburn is a valuable contribution to the treatment of an extremely prevalent disorder. This book discusses many lifestyle factors that may be modified. Also included is a comprehensive dietary section suggesting many measures to decrease symptoms. Authored by a physician and registered dietitian, this book is a well written, practical guide for all heartburn suffers.

Diane D. Hester, MS, R.D. C.N.S.D.
Clinical Nutrition Manager
Stanford University Medical Center and Lucile Packard Children's
Hospital at Stanford

I had acid reflux for many years. The information in this book gave me relief within a few weeks. That acid is pretty powerful stuff. I could never go back to my original lifestyle without having heartburn, cough, and a hoarse voice.

Mr. Walter Carter
Sunnyvale California

I had trouble with coughing and throat clearing. The advice that I found in this book, with respect to the foods I eat and the way I sleep, helped my symptoms a great deal. My wife even likes sleeping with the head of the bed elevated.

Mr. Elijah Nelson
Monterey California

the **AUTHOR**

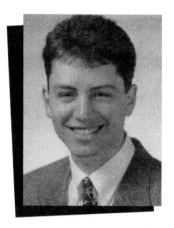

David S. Utley, M.D. attended Harvard Medical School and then entered the residency training program in otolaryngology-head and neck surgery at Stanford University Hospital. He was interested by the large number of patients seen in the ear, nose and throat clinic who reported complaints related to heartburn and the effects of refluxed stomach acid on the structures in the throat.

Further study revealed heartburn and reflux of stomach acid to be a universal problem. Millions of people are seen yearly in clinics across the country. Physicians in nearly every medical specialty surveyed report seeing patients with heartburn symptoms.

Physician specialists who manage heartburn symptoms include:

- Endocrinologists
- Emergency Medicine Physicians
- Family Practitioners
- Gastroenterologist (digestion)
- Geriatrics (elderly)
- Internal Medicine Physicians
- Obstetricians
- Otolaryngologists (ear, nose and throat)
- Pediatricians (children)
- Psychiatrists
- Pulmonologists
- Radiation Oncologists
- Rheumatologists

Most patients with complaints of heartburn and related symptoms are treated with medications. (These include antacid preparations and anti-acid drugs like Zantac®.) Fewer are treated with simple, effective, common-sense lifestyle changes. While some individuals have a definite need for pharmacological therapy, the medical literature states that the majority of heartburn / reflux suffers can be successfully treated without medication. The evolving U.S. health care system also mandates simple, effective measures before using expensive drugs.

This book will take you through the education process for learning about heartburn and reflux and will then give you the proper steps to take to eliminate or reduce your symptoms. Consult your primary care physician regarding your symptoms after having read this book. If your symptoms persist, you may need therapy and referral to a specialist.

Credits:

Kathryn M. Utley, MS, RD

Kathryn has a Master's in Clinical Nutrition and works as a nutritionist in the Neonatal Intensive Care Unit at the Lucile Salter Packard Children's Hospital at Stanford. She developed the chapters in this book addressing the role of nutrition in treating Gastroesophageal Reflux Disease.

James R. Weber

James is a Cleveland-based graphic designer. He is the art director for two regional publications. His freelance work includes logo design, corporate identity and book design.

Sheryl L. Lewin

Sheryl is a Stanford medical student with an architectural background. She provided the anatomical art work.

table of CONTENTS

America's **BURNING** **HEALTH** *problem*

There are thousands of different medical problems managed by physicians and endured by individuals like yourself. You may be surprised to find that one of these health problems affects over one hundred million people in this country. You may be even more surprised to find that you may have some of the symptoms and complaints of this process.

One of America's most common health problems is Gastroesophageal Reflux Disease or GERD. What is reflux? Gastroesophageal reflux occurs when stomach acids and digestive enzymes flow backwards into the throat causing symptoms of heartburn and sore throat. These symptoms are the most common complaints seen by physicians in this country.

Reflux has a significant economic impact. Americans spend $3 billion annually on stomach-acid reducing prescription drugs. Another $600 million is spent on over-the-counter antacid medications.

When considering all of America's minor and major illnesses which produce significant symptoms and have the potential to cause injury, gastroesophageal reflux disease affects an enormous number of people.

Facts

United States Population	**248 Million**
Individuals with Reflux symptoms monthly	**75-100 Million**
Individuals with Reflux symptoms on a daily basis	**24 Million**
Individuals taking antacids for Reflux	**67 Million**
Adults with Asthma	**12 Million**
Asthmatic adults who have reflux which worsens their asthma	**6 Million**

gastroesophageal
REFLUX *disease*

You might now ask, "Reflux certainly is a common problem. How do I know if I have this problem too?"

Reflux disease affects many people and it does so by causing a wide variety of symptoms and complaints. Many people have reflux symptoms and are never told what is causing their symptoms. The following is a list of the many ways in which reflux disease can cause discomfort.

Are you currently experiencing any of these symptoms?

- Heartburn
- Difficulty Swallowing
- Sour Taste in the Mouth with Heartburn
- Sour Taste in the Mouth when Lying Flat
- Painful Swallowing
- Indigestion
- Excessive Belching

- Hoarseness
- Persistently Sore Throat
- Chronic Cough
- Tickle in the Throat
- Asthma
- Frequent Lung Infections (children, elderly)
- Waterbrash - Excessive Salivation Caused by Reflux
- Throat Clearing

Individuals with reflux disease may have one or many of these symptoms. It is a good idea to visit your family physician to discuss any particular symptoms on this list that you may be experiencing. You may benefit from treatment or a referral to a specialist.

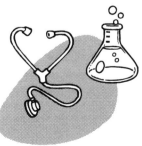

what are the *MOST COMMON SYMPTOMS OF* reflux disease?

The number one complaint among all people with reflux disease is heartburn. This usually occur after eating a big meal or while lying flat.

Between 75 and 125 million people in the United States have reflux which becomes symptomatic at least once or twice per month. Most of these individuals have heartburn as their number one complaint. Most people treat their discomfort with over-the-counter antacid preparations and never enlist the help of their physician for diagnosis or therapy.

Each year about 15 million of these individuals with heartburn visit their family physician or a medical specialist for help. Which specialists are most often called upon to treat reflux symptoms?

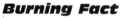

Burning Fact

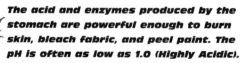

The acid and enzymes produced by the stomach are powerful enough to burn skin, bleach fabric, and peel paint. The pH is often as low as 1.0 (Highly Acidic).

Gastroenterologists (digestion doctors) treat reflux everyday. They report that their patients have heartburn as the number one complaint. Cough is the second most common.

Ear, nose, and throat physicians also treat reflux effectively, seeing patients with reflux complaints about as frequently as the gastroenterologist. Because of the nature of the specialty, these patients report throat irritation as the most common symptom. Hoarse voice ranks as number two.

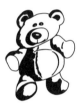

Pediatricians treat many children with reflux disease as well. The number one pediatric symptom is frequent regurgitation of food (vomiting). The number two complaint is recurrent lung infections.

It is important to remember... You do not have to have heartburn to have reflux. Over half of individuals with reflux of stomach contents into the esophagus report they never experience heartburn. Most of these people had one or more of the other symptoms mentioned in the previous section. Your family physician or medical specialist can help you determine what process is causing your particular symptoms.

the *STOMACH*

The stomach acts as a reservoir for foods and liquids.

The stomach temporarily stores the food and liquid while digestion takes place in the intestines further downstream. As room becomes available in the intestines, the contents of the stomach are slowly released for digestion.

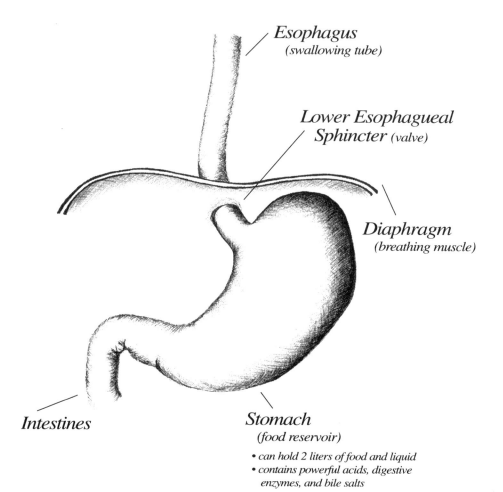

Esophagus
(swallowing tube)

Lower Esophagueal Sphincter (valve)

Diaphragm
(breathing muscle)

Intestines

Stomach
(food reservoir)
- *can hold 2 liters of food and liquid*
- *contains powerful acids, digestive enzymes, and bile salts*

the *ESOPHAGUS*

The esophagus is the swallowing tube which connects your mouth and throat to your stomach. It is a muscular tube which helps to propel food and liquids into the stomach.

At the junction of the esophagus and stomach, there is a one-way valve called the lower esophageal sphincter. This valve is often called the LES for short. It will be refered to frequently in this book as the LES valve.

The LES valve opens briefly during swallowing to permit food to enter the stomach. The LES valve then snaps shut helping to prevent stomach contents from squirting back up into the esophagus, mouth and throat.

If the LES valve is faulty or if it relaxes when it shouldn't, stomach contents will squirt back into the esophagus. This is called gastroesophageal reflux.

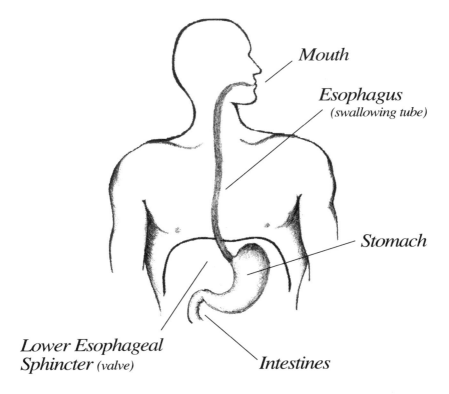

Mouth

Esophagus
(swallowing tube)

Stomach

Lower Esophageal
Sphincter *(valve)*

Intestines

what is
GASTROESOPHAGEAL
reflux disease?

The word Gastroesophageal refers to the stomach (Gastro) and the swallowing tube (Esophageal.)

The word Reflux is from Latin, Fluere (to flow) and Re (backwards.)

Gastroesophageal Reflux = The back flow of stomach contents into the esophagus frequently causing uncomfortable symptoms.

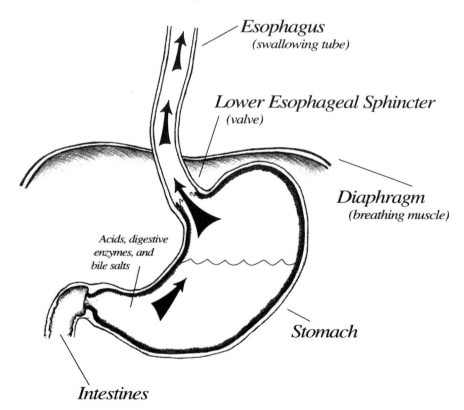

Esophagus
(swallowing tube)

Lower Esophageal Sphincter
(valve)

Diaphragm
(breathing muscle)

Acids, digestive enzymes, and bile salts

Stomach

Intestines

what goes **INTO** **THE STOMACH** *everyday?*

The average American will consume about four liters of fluid and food in one day.

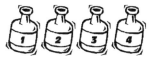

Add an additional two liters of digestive juices produced by the mouth and throat.

Add to that an additional five liters of digestive juices produced by the stomach every day, essential to digestion.

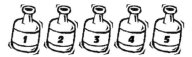

This totals eleven liters of fluid, food and digestive juices that the stomach stores, mixes and sends downstream to the intestines everyday. That's over three gallons!

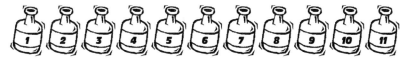

The stomach juices are very irritating to the esophagus because they contain powerful acids needed for digestion. To give you two examples, if you were to spill these acids on your skin, you would sustain quite a chemical burn. If you were to spill these acids on your carpet, you would bleach the color and probably end up with a hole in the material. From this analogy you can imagine that the esophagus must become very irritated if exposed to frequent acid reflux episodes.

why doesn't the **STOMACH** **GET BURNED** by these acids?

The stomach is protected on the inside by a special coating. In most people this protective layer doesn't allow the acid to harm the stomach lining.

The esophagus, however, does not have this same protective layer and is easily burned by the acid. If the LES valve between the esophagus and stomach malfunctions, the esophagus is exposed to the stomach acid frequently. When this happens, patients experience symptoms, like heartburn, as mentioned in the previous section. If the exposure to acid is prolonged and your heartburn is left untreated, the esophagus can become severely irritated or eroded. These severe complications of reflux require careful management by a gastroenterologist (digestion doctor).

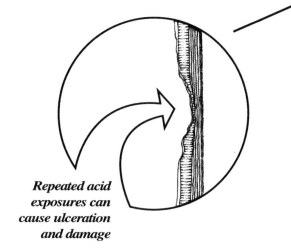

Repeated acid exposures can cause ulceration and damage

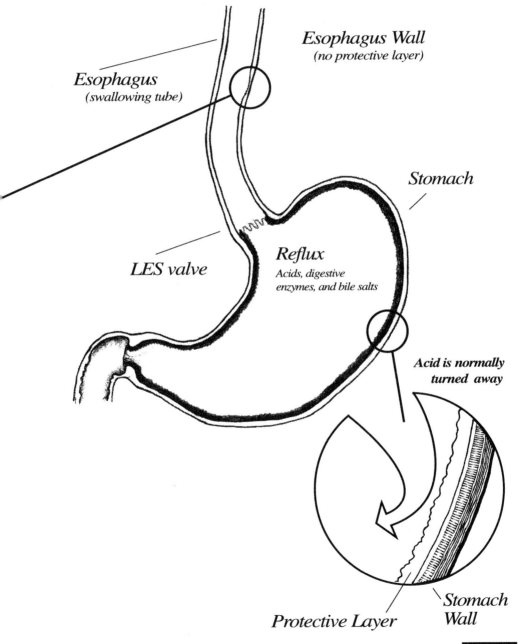

Esophagus Wall
(no protective layer)

Esophagus
(swallowing tube)

Stomach

LES valve

Reflux
Acids, digestive
enzymes, and bile salts

Acid is normally
turned away

Protective Layer

Stomach
Wall

what are the *EVENTS* **WHICH TAKE PLACE** *during* *a reflux* **EPISODE** ?

Research physicians and scientists have determined that reflux will occur when any one of the following events takes place:

1. The LES valve between the stomach and esophagus relaxes for a moment and allows the stomach acids to squirt back up into the esophagus.

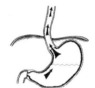

2. The LES valve is faulty or is injured by a long history of reflux exposure. In this case the LES valve is never able to tightly seal off the stomach acids from reaching the esophagus.

3. The person strains, bends over, or eats a huge meal which increases the pressure in the stomach. Just like water in a water balloon, the contents of the stomach become more likely to reflux into the esophagus if there is increased pressure on the outside of the stomach.

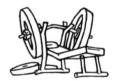

The most common reason for reflux is relaxation of the protective LES valve (see item 1 above). Scientists have shown that even in unaffected persons, the valve relaxes approximately two times per hour.

With this in mind, it's interesting to know that everyone has times throughout the day when stomach contents reflux into the esophagus. These occur while the LES valve is taking a "relaxation break" every 30 minutes.

So if everyone has hourly reflux events (that's 250 million people in the U.S.), why isn't everyone suffering from the symptoms of reflux, heartburn and sore throats? The answer relates to how well the esophagus can handle the reflux. (This is described in the next section).

everyone refluxes

DURING THE DAY
BUT NOT *everyone has symptoms*

A brief reflux of acid into the healthy esophagus is usually not noticed by most individuals. The acid is quickly re-swallowed in about two gulps and then saliva from the mouth neutralizes the acid. The process of swallowing clears the acid in about 30 seconds. It then takes up to 5 minutes to neutralize the small amount of residual acid with saliva. The healthy esophagus can endure many of these brief episodes without injury.

A problem arises when the reflux events become either more frequent or more prolonged. More frequent reflux episodes may be the result of overeating, straining, pregnancy, or foods which cause reflux. These topics will be explained in the next section.

More prolonged episodes of reflux may be the result of impaired swallowing mechanisms, decreased saliva production, or medication use. These topics will also be explained in the next section.

As reflux events become more frequent and prolonged, the esophagus may not be able to resist injury by the acids and enzymes of the stomach. The lining of the esophagus becomes irritated, red, swollen, or ulcerated, like your hands after doing heavy garden work. At this point, the person begins having more severe symptoms of burning and discomfort.

Burning Fact

Aspirin, non-steroidal anti-inflammatory medicines, and smoking weaken the protective lining of the stomach, resulting in a greater likelihood of developing gastritis and ulceration.

once the *ESOPHAGUS* *BECOMES* irritated, the following *MAY OCCUR*

1. The LES valve begins to malfunction even further. The acid may then reflux even more easily.

2. The irritation and swelling in the esophagus make it more sensitive to acid, just as blisters on your hands become more sensitive to the touch. Now each reflux event is experienced as pain, heartburn, or discomfort.

3. Reflux becomes more severe and frequent, beginning to affect other areas like the throat and voice box. Symptoms now may include hoarseness and sore throat.

4. The esophagus also may lose some of its natural acid protective mechanisms, making it even more susceptible to permanent damage.

Burning Fact

Five million (5,000,000) cells that line the stomach die every minute. The dead cells are released into the stomach and intestine where they are digested. The lining of the stomach is entirely renewed every 3 days!

can reflux **CAUSE** **PERMANENT** damage?

In the most severe cases, reflux can cause permanent and debilitating injury to the esophagus if not recognized and treated early. Gastroesophageal reflux is a process which presents a variety of symptoms and a spectrum of severity.

People at the mild end of the spectrum will be unlikely to develop any long-term problems from their occasional reflux events. These people with mild symptoms should practice the lifestyle changes mentioned later in this book to prevent worsening of symptoms. Most individuals who have mild reflux symptoms are easily treated with lifestyle management and occasional over-the-counter antacid preparations. We recommend enlisting the care of your physician if you have any questions regarding this process.

At the more severe end of the spectrum, the patient with frequent reflux episodes and persistent symptoms will need more intensive therapy by a physician. A proper medical work-up is warranted for these individuals to ensure that reflux is indeed the cause of their symptoms. These individuals may also need medication for a period of time to initiate the healing process. If you have persistent symptoms, it is your responsibility to visit your primary care physician for proper management. An appropriate referral may be made to a gastroenterologist or an otolaryngologist based on the location of your symptoms.

People at the more severe end of the spectrum definitely have a higher risk of developing long-term complications from their reflux disease. The following is a comprehensive list of the many complications that may be seen with untreated, severe reflux.

- Esophageal Ulceration
- Voice Box Growths, Swelling
- Esophageal Stricture
- Narrowing of the Trachea (windpipe)
- Barrett's Esophagus

- Cancer of the Voice Box
- Cancer of the Esophagus
- Chronic Lung Infections
- Severe Swallowing Difficulty
- Asthma that becomes worse with Reflux

Burning Fact

A man from Grenoble, France is known as "Mr.-Eat-anything." In his lifetime he has eaten 2 shopping carts, 10 bicycles, 7 TV sets, 6 chandeliers, a Cessna airplane, and a computer. Surprisingly, he denies having heartburn.

what factors **IN MY** **LIFESTYLE** are contributing to my **REFLUX** ?

The following is the most up to date, scientifically-based list of all of the lifestyle and dietary factors that may either cause or contribute to gastroesophageal reflux disease.

- Late-Night Eating
- Hiatal Hernias
- Coffee and Tea Consumption
- Tomatoes, Citrus, and Spicy Foods
- Chocolate Consumption
- Soda Consumption
- High-fat Foods
- Excess Body Weight
- Tight Clothing Around the Mid-section
- Increased Age (over 60)
- Tobacco Use
- Bending, Squatting or Straining
- Alcohol Consumption
- Eating Huge meals
- Spearmint and Peppermint
- Stressful Lifestyles
- Belching and Burping
- Competitive Athletics

If any of these factors affect you, refer to the next section which will discuss why each factor makes reflux worse, and make recommendations on how to alleviate the symptoms.

late-night EATING

In today's busy world, most people find there are just not enough hours in the day. Often people find themselves eating dinner at 8 or 9 p.m. and heading off to bed shortly thereafter with a full belly.

Lying flat with a full stomach increases your chance for having a reflux event. The volume of acid in the stomach will be higher after a meal. The higher acid content means that each reflux event will have a greater chance of burning and irritating the esophagus. The large volume of food in the stomach also makes it more likely for food and acid to squirt back up into the esophagus.

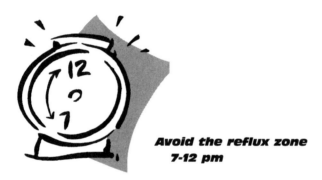

**Avoid the reflux zone
7-12 pm**

When you lie flat in bed, your esophagus is horizontal. This means your mouth and stomach are at the same level. Any acid that is refluxed in this position will tend to remain in the esophagus longer before it is cleared back into the stomach. Why? Because gravity is not working in your favor and because swallowing isn't effective during sleep. Salivation also decreases at night, which reduces the ability to neutralize refluxed acid. This can lead to uncomfortable symptoms.

Recommendations

1. Elevate the head of your bed (see appendix page 93). This allows gravity to work in your favor to clear refluxed acid out of your esophagus. Sleeping with one or two extra pillows will not reduce reflux events, since the stomach and esophagus remain horizontal when pillows are placed under the head.

2. Schedule your evening meal at least three to four hours before retiring to bed. Avoid the reflux zone.

3. Avoid snacks and liquids before retiring.

4. Observe the other lifestyle management recommendations reviewed in his manual.

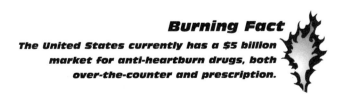

Burning Fact
The United States currently has a $5 billion market for anti-heartburn drugs, both over-the-counter and prescription.

hiatal **HERNIA**

A hiatal hernia occurs when the connection of the esophagus and stomach slides up through the diaphragm muscle opening. This is a common problem and seems to be even more common in people over the age of 60.

If you have been told you have a hiatal hernia, you do not automatically have gastroesophageal reflux disease. There are many people with a hiatal hernia who have no symptoms of reflux. However, most studies show an association between hiatal hernia and reflux disease. This means people with a hiatal hernia have a higher chance of having reflux and esophageal irritation than people without a hiatal hernia.

Recommendations

1. There is no medication that can cure hiatal hernia. Medication may be used, however, to reduce acid production and reduce your reflux symptoms. Although surgery is the only way to totally correct hiatal hernia, most individual's symptoms of reflux can be treated with lifestyle management and occasional medication. Surgery should be considered for those individuals with severe, potentially damaging, intractable reflux disease.

2. Elevate the head of your bed.

3. Observe all of the lifestyle recommendations reviewed in this manual.

coffee and *TEA* CONSUMPTION

America's favorite beverages for waking up and socializing are coffee and tea. These both worsen reflux symptoms and may actually cause reflux in some people. Researchers initially felt that the caffeine and other caffeine-like substances reduced the ability of the LES valve to function properly. This is why many individuals were told to switch to decaffeinated products to reduce reflux.

Now it appears that coffee and tea act directly, independent of the presence of caffeine to irritate the esophagus lining and to increase the amount of acid produced in the stomach. The irritation and increased acid production combine to worsen or cause reflux disease. Decaffeinated products often have the same effects.

Other similar foods may act in the same way to worsen or cause reflux disease. These include carbonated beverages (colas, beers), citrus fruits, tomatos, and even raw onions. Colas are a triple whammy with caffeine, carbonation and acid pH, all of which directly irritate the esophagus.

Recommendations

1. Avoid these foods! That's easy to say, but giving up your morning coffee may be next to impossible. A more workable suggestion could be to decrease your intake of these beverages and to consume them early in the day.
2. You may also want to try drinking weaker coffee and tea. Follow such beverages with a glass of water and/or a tablespoon of antacid.
3. Observe the other lifestyle management recommendations reviewed in this manual.

tomatoes, citrus and **SPICY FOODS**

These acidic or spicy foods are considered by many reflux sufferers to be a chief cause of their heartburn symptoms. In fact, many of our patients able to name a single food in these categories which eaten, will send them running for the antacid bottle.

the list includes:

- Any tomato product; pizza, spaghetti, sauced tomatoes, etc.
- Citrus fruits and juices: oranges, pineapple, guava, grapefruit
- Onions: especially raw onions
- Spicy foods: mexican food, hot chinese food, salsa cayenne pepper, chile peppers, hot sauces

The medical literature does not show that any of these foods directly cause reflux. However, the anecdotal evidence is clear. These foods can make certain people very uncomfortable. The recommendations here are to avoid the offending foods, and use antacids after consuming these foods.

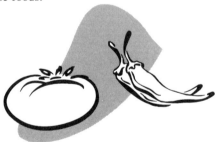

Burning Fact

The "heat" in a chile pepper is due to the substance capsaicin. Each type of pepper has a different level of heat, as measured by the Scoville Organoleptic Test. The most mild on the list is the bell pepper with a rating of zero. Compare this to the world's most incendiary and pungent chile pepper, the habanero, with a rating of 300,000!

CHOCOLATE consumption

Chocolate lovers prepare yourselves. Chocolate has been shown with little doubt to cause reflux events in a variety of ways. Chocolate has a very high fat content which slows the emptying of the stomach and relaxes the LES valve. There is also a caffeine-like substance in chocolate which has been shown to further loosen the strength of the LES valve.

Recommendations

1. Chocolate lovers, you may not like hearing this one. If you are suffering from symptoms of reflux disease, avoiding chocolate will clearly improve your symptoms.

2. Try lower fat chocolate brands or chocolate substitutes.

3. Follow chocolate with a tablespoon of antacid one hour after eating.

4. Observe the other lifestyle management recommendations reviewed in this manual.

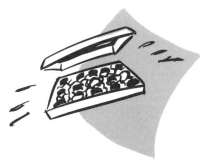

SODA consumption

University students and business people often complain about severe heartburn. Most of these people are young and fit. They often do not have many of the obvious risk factors for reflux disease. However, when these people are asked about their cola (caffeine containing sodas) intake, it's often learned they will drink between 3 and 5 cans per day. The average diet cola intake in the symptomatic patients is 45 ounces a day (almost 4 cans).

Caffeinated colas should be considered a triple whammy for reflux sufferers. The carbonation and acidity irritate the esophagus directly on the way down. The stomach's acid production increases dramatically after drinking a caffeinated cola / soda. The carbonation and the caffeine act together to increase reflux events; carbonation causes belching and caffeine relaxes the LES valve.

Recommendations

1. Cimit soda intake.
2. Change to clear caffeine-free sodas.
3. Substitute other beverages such as non-acidic fruit juices or caffeine-free iced teas.
4. Observe the other lifestyle management recommendations reviewed in this manual.

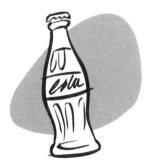

high-fat *FOODS*

High-fat foods have been shown unequivocally to lower the strength of the LES valve. This significantly increases the number of times that reflux occurs for up to three hours after the fatty meals. The fat in the food releases a hormone from the stomach called CCK which loosens the LES valve.

A second factor with high-fat foods is that the fat slows the rate at which the stomach can empty (fat is more difficult to digest). Since the stomach stays fuller for a longer period of time, the likelihood of reflux is much higher. This would be very likely to cause reflux if you were lying flat with a belly full of a fatty meal.

Recommendations

1. Refer to the section on nutrition (page 72).
2. Obtain an American Heart Association approved cookbook with ideas for heart-healthy low-fat meals.
3. Reduce the obvious fats in your diet first such as butter and margarine, junk foods, doughnuts and pastries, etc. Once these have been recognized, you can move on to examining your diet for many of the hidden fats. An American Heart Association cookbook will be quite helpful in identifying fat in your diet.
4. Observe the other lifestyle management recommendations reviewed in this manual.

Burning Fact

In 1995 United States consumers ate 5 billion pounds of snack food (over 20 pounds each) and 34 billion pounds of sugar (over 120 pounds each).

excess BODY WEIGHT

People who are more than ten to twenty percent heavier than their ideal body weight (see appendix chart to determine your own ideal body weight, page 95) will be more susceptible to having reflux disease. Medical research has never conclusively shown that the overweight person's LES valve malfunctions. However, it is clear from the medical literature that the excess weight in the belly places more pressure on the stomach and worsens reflux when the LES valve loosens normally about fifty times per day. Each reflux episode then has the potential to contain a higher volume of stomach contents, which means more acid and more irritation.

Recommendations

1. See your physician to start a weight loss program today. Remember, if you are above your ideal body weight, even a modest amount of weight loss coupled with a healthy anti-reflux menu and lifestyle will dramatically reduce your reflux symptoms.

2. Refer to page 82 for information on low-fat foods and recipes.

3. Elevate the head of your bed.

4. Observe the other lifestyle management recommendations reviewed in this manual.

Burning Fact

40% of the United States adult population is estimated to be overweight. This has increased by about 10% since 1978.

tight **CLOTHING**
AROUND *the midsection*

Tight belts or pants, girdles, support hose, etc. all place pressure on the belly and subsequently on the stomach. Any pressure on the belly will certainly lead to more severe reflux episodes when the LES valve relaxes over the course of the day and night.

Recommendations

1. Loosen the belt and lose the tight stuff!

2. Wear loose night clothing. Tight bed clothes around the belly while lying flat will exacerbate reflux symptoms. Try loose boxers, big nightshirts, etc.

3. Observe the other lifestyle management recommendations reviewed in this manual.

Burning Fact

The largest amount of body weight ever lost while dieting is 920 pounds, when a man slimmed down from 1396 to 476 pounds over 16 months.

increased **AGE** *(over 60)*

While gastroesophageal reflux is extremely common in all age groups, people over the age of 60 are particularly susceptible to the effects of reflux. This is due to a number of changes in the body as one grows older as well as to the variety of medications that are prescribed for this age group.

Studies have shown the following findings in people over the age of 60 that may lead to reflux disease or to the delay in treatment of reflux disease:

- Decrease in LES valve protective muscle tone with the normal aging process.
- Decreased saliva production. Saliva is needed to neutralize and wash away refluxed acid.
- Decreased motility of the esophagus. This movement is needed to swallow refluxed acid.
- Slowed emptying of the stomach after meals, especially in persons with diabetes.
- Medications often necessary in persons over the age of 60 may worsen reflux (See the following section on medications and reflux on page 51).
- People in this age group are often brave and stoic when it comes to bothersome symptoms. For this reason, reflux in this group often goes undetected by the person's physician until irritation or damage to the esophagus has started.

Burning Fact

In 1990, there were 35,808 centarians living in the United States (people over 100 years of age).

Recommendations

1. Observe strict anti-reflux precautions.

2. Elevate the head of your bed.

3. Ask your physician about any changes in your medication regimen that could be made to lessen your risk for reflux. Show your physician the medication list in this book.

4. Consume adequate fluids to optimize saliva production. Chewing gum, candies and lozenges also promote salivation.

5. Observe the other lifestyle management recommendations reviewed in this manual.

Burning Fact

People over the age of 65 make up only 12% of the United States population, (31.7 million), yet buy 34% of prescription drugs. This age group is particularly likely to develop heartburn and reflux.

TOBACCO use

Tobacco use of any kind has a direct effect on the LES valve by decreasing the valve's ability to maintain a one-way route from the esophagus to the stomach. Nicotine may be the substance which causes dysfunction of the LES valve. It also increases the number of reflux events per day and decreases the protective barrier on the esophagus lining. Nicotine also increases acid production in the stomach so that each reflux event has a higher potential for injuring the esophagus.

Some patients with gastroesophageal reflux disease require a temporary course of anti-acid medications called H-2 blockers prescribed by their physician. These medications reduce acid production and allow esophageal healing to begin. Tobacco products actually interfere with the medication's effect. This is usually not recognized by the patient or physician and results in a longer, more expensive course of medication therapy.

Therefore, cigarettes, cigars, pipes, chewing tobacco, snuff, etc. increase the number of reflux events, make the esophagus more susceptible to injury, increase acid production, and interfere with many of the prescribed anti-acid medications.

Nicotine gum and nicotine patches may have the same effects as tobacco on reflux disease and should only be used temporarily under the observation of your physician.

Recommendations

1. Smoking cessation (tobacco cessation) is the only alternative for improving the symptoms of reflux. There are many professional and peer groups to help you in this very difficult task. (see appendix for a listing of these groups, page 94)

2. Ask your physician for counselling regarding tobacco cessation. Inquire about temporary medications which can help

3. Observe the other lifestyle management recommendations reviewed in this manual.

bending, squatting, **STRAINING**

Any process which increases the pressure on the stomach will encourage reflux events. Add the above "bending, squatting and straining" to the list of:

- Tight clothing around the midsection
- Huge meals, especially at night
- Being overweight

Remember that most reflux occurs when the LES valve spontaneously relaxes a number of times throughout the day. A straining effort can actually overcome a normally functioning LES valve and can force acid through the valve into the esophagus. Imagine if the straining episode occurred while the LES valve was taking a relaxation break. The reflux event would be even more severe.

Examples of these "bending, squatting, straining" movements are:

- Tying your shoelaces
- Lifting heavy objects
- Straining to have a bowel movement
- Coughing
- Sneezing

Recommendations

1. Avoid movements and positions in your life which require straining.

2. Ask your physician or pharmacist for a stool softener or laxative.

3. Increase the fiber in your diet.

4. Observe general anti-reflux precautions in this book.

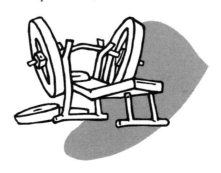

ALCOHOL *consumption*

Alcohol includes beer, wine, and liquor. Intake of alcohol, especially when consumed within four hours of retiring to bed, dramatically increases the acid production in the stomach. It also acts directly on the LES valve, reducing the valve's ability to function normally. These two factors combine to cause more frequent reflux events, each with a higher concentration of acid. If that's not enough, alcohol also directly irritates the esophageal lining and makes it much more susceptible to acid injury. It may also delay emptying of the stomach.

Alcohol has a sedative effect which is magnified when you fall asleep. Normally a reflux event while sleeping will partly arouse you enough for your swallowing mechanism to "wake up" and take care of the acid. Alcohol and other sedatives don't allow the person or the swallowing mechanism to wake up properly. This allows the acid to remain in the esophagus for a long period of time, as long as 45 minutes, causing injury to the esophagus. Remember, while lying flat you do not have gravity working with you to clear the acid unless you elevate the head of your bed.

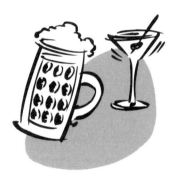

Lastly, alcohol in excess has a strong causative association with major cancers of the mouth, throat, esophagus and voice box. When combined with tobacco products, the risk of cancer increases twenty-fold. This means that if you smoke tobacco and drink alcohol, you have a twenty times higher risk of developing a cancer of the head and neck than if you avoid tobacco and alcohol.

Recommendations

1. Limit alcohol in general and avoid entirely four hours before retiring to bed. This will improve your comfort with respect to reflux.

2. Drink alcohol in moderation or eliminate to improve your overall health and well being.

3. General reflux precautions should always be employed, including elevating the head of your bed.

4. Observe the anti-reflux precautions mentioned in this manual.

Burning Fact

1.7 billion pounds of tobacco were produced in the United States last year, about 7 pounds for every U.S. citizen.

huge MEALS

If you are a two- or three-meal per day person with each of these meals being rather large, you may be setting yourself up for worsened symptoms of reflux disease. It especially applies to you if your last meal of the day is your biggest of the day and if it is consumed just before retiring to bed. A huge meal will obviously increase the pressure inside the stomach. This will work to drive acid back up into the esophagus.

Eating a big meal and then lying flat is a double whammy. The food in the stomach increases pressure and causes reflux. Lying flat prevents gravity from working in your favor and allows the acid to lie in the esophagus for longer periods of time.

Recommendations

1. Seneral anti-reflux precautions including elevating the head of the bed.
2. Increase the number of meals per day to five or six, while decreasing the size of each meal to one half or less of the usual size.
3. Make your last meal of the day your smallest.
4. Eat your last meal of the day at least three hours before retiring to bed.
5. Observe standard anti-reflux precautions in this manual.

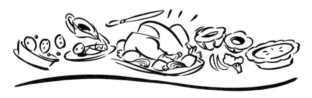

Burning Fact

Every year on the day before Lent, the church-goers in Ponti, Italy prepare and eat a 1000 egg omelet, the largest omelet and meal on record.

spearmint and **PEPPERMINT**

Spearmint and peppermint are members of the carminative family, compounds which have clearly been shown in medical research to worsen gastroesophageal reflux by reducing the function of the LES valve.

There are reports of patients who complained of reflux discomfort for months and months. These patients were not helped by any lifestyle modifications or medications. Finally a physician or a knowledgeable family member suggested eliminating all spearmint and peppermint from their diet. This would include mints, certain candies, gums, and spices. Within one week these patients were remarkably improved.

Any candy, gum or lozenge that is spearmint or peppermint free will actually help to clear acid from the esophagus. This occurs by stimulation of saliva production in the mouth which washes out and neutralizes acid in the esophagus.

Recommendations

1. Eliminate all spearmint and peppermint products.

2. Substitute plain gums, cinnamon gums/candies, lozenges, etc. for your previous mint-containing products.

Burning Fact
Any gum or lozenge which promotes saliva production will help to neutralize acid within the esophagus after a reflux event.

45

stressful LIFESTYLE

Ask anyone in the 1990s if their life is stressed out and you will find that most will say YES!

Stress comes from:

- Long hours of work either in or out of the home
- Late-night dinners
- Excessive coffee consumption
- Lack of sleep
- Fast food
- Financial worries
- Job woes
- Retiring to bed late
- Managing a busy family
- Getting up very early
- Commuting in heavy traffic
- Perfectionism
- Competition
- Feeling a need to control situations
- Feeling a need to please everyone

Experts in the field of stress management explain that an individual must identify the particular aspects of his or her life which are most likely to be the stress causing agents. The list above includes examples, but you may have many other reasons to feel anxious, irritable, as stress.

Many of these stressors have been noted to increase the number of reflux events and will worsen your symptoms. Stress in general will increase the amount of acid produced by the stomach.

Stress can also cause insomnia, eating disorders, addiction, and reduced immunity.

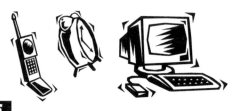

Recommendations

1. Stress experts list the following suggestions to reduce stress.
  - Reduce coffee consumption
  - Engage in regular exercise
  - Start relaxation / meditation classes
  - Increase sleep time, including an occasional nap
  - Take time outs and leisure breaks
  - Have realistic expectations, as unattainable goals not met resulting in frustration.
  - Reframe the situation — this is to put things into perspective. Say to yourself, "How bad is this, really? Am I stressed over something that really isn't that big of a deal?
  - Inject humor whenever possible. Smile at rude people, they'll hate it.
  - Go shopping!
  - Get a massage!
  - Surround yourself with supportive people so you can ventilate your frustrations.
  - Give up the attitudes of perfectionism, people pleasing, and need to control everything around you.
  - Avoid unnecessary competition
  - Prioritize the things you need to do today.

2. Follow the general anti-reflux precautions including elevating the head of the bed.

3. Start a program today to reduce the stress in your life. This program could include walking after dinner, reading before going to bed, setting aside time to listen to classical music in the evenings, or joining a health club.

4. Read books on the subject of effectively dealing with stress.

5. Start a daily exercise program. This can be any form of exercise, walking, aerobics, jogging, swimming, etc. The importance of exercising daily to reduce stress can not be over emphasized. Remember, you don't have to workout vigorously to relieve stress. Consult with your doctor before beginning any workout program.

belching and **BURPING**

One thing known about belching is that there is no such thing as a dry belch. If you belch air and gas, you simultaneously reflux stomach contents and acid into your esophagus. A healthy belch is normal and helps to relieve gas pressure in the stomach. Some people, however, encourage themselves to belch frequently and will occasionally induce belching by swallowing air. This may not be healthy.

Each time a belch occurs, the LES valve must relax to allow air to pass from the stomach into the esophagus. Acid will move with the gas or will reflux afterwards when the LES valve is still not tight.

Recommendations

1. Do not induce belching by swallowing air.
2. Avoid carbonated beverages, especially before going to bed.
3. Elevate the head of your bed.
4. Try one of the over-the-counter products labelled antacid/anti-gas. These products contain simethicone, which reduces gas.
5. Observe anti-reflux precautions in this manual.

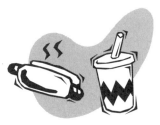

Burning Fact

In 1994, a 6 year-old first grader burped 844 consecutive times while his classmates counted and cheered him on. A new worlds record!

competitive ATHLETICS

You would not think that a competitive athlete would be susceptible to reflux disease, but it may be quite common in this group. "Competitive athlete" in this context implies an individual who is training for more than just fitness, has a particular race or competition in mind, and trains at least 5-10 hours per week.

Serious athletes are susceptible to reflux for the following reasons:
- The LES has been shown to relax somewhat during exercise
- Highly competitive athletes may also be engaging in weight training and sit-ups during which time there is an increase in the abdominal pressure. This may increase reflux.
- Competitive athletes are generally busy individuals with erratic schedules. This may necessitate late-night meals and a full belly upon retiring to bed.
- These athletes are often trying to eat a large volume of food to replenish the huge amount of calories that they expend everyday working out. Sometimes this means a second dinner at late hours. This will also lead to retiring to bed with a full belly.

Before anyone reads this and says, "Athletes get reflux, so I'm definitely not going to start my exercise program," remember that this applies to serious athletes, not weekend warriors. If you need to begin exercising, the benefits that you will derive from weight loss and increased activity will far outweigh any reflux you might cause by exercising. So put on your shoes and get out there!

Recommendations

1. Observe the standard anti-reflux precautions including elevating the head of your bed.
2. Limit evening meals to three or more hours prior to bed time.

Burning Fact

The progesterone in many contraceptive preparations can also worsen or cause reflux symptoms in some women by relaxing the LES valve.

MEDICAL problems
which lead to
REFLUX SYMPTOMS

The previous section reviewed the factors in a persons lifestyle which may be influencing or causing reflux symptoms. An individual has some control over most of these factors.

This section reviews processes over which we have less control. This will include four types of situations in which an underlying illness or medication may be contributing to the symptoms of reflux. The four categories include:

1. Asthma
2. Pregnancy
3. Decreased saliva production
4. Increased stomach acid production
5. Swallowing disorders
6. Conditions in which the stomach empties more slowly than normal
7. Medications that can worsen reflux

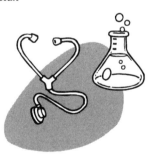

ASTHMA

It has been estimated that twelve million adults in the United States suffer from asthma. Of these, between five and eight million adults have symptomatic reflux disease detectable by traditional studies for reflux (pH probe study).

The evidence shows that reflux of acid into the esophagus triggers a nerve reflex which causes constriction of the small airways of the lungs. What's the result? Worsened asthma and a need for more frequent asthma medication.

Reflux of acid into the esophagus frequently reaches as high as the voice box and mouth. Sometimes the acid enters the wind pipe and lungs, an event called aspiration. This causes a direct irritation that causes the airways to constrict. What's the result? Again, worsened asthma and a need for more frequent asthma medication.

Furthermore, asthma medication such as theophylline, beta adrenergic inhalers, and oral agents have been shown to decrease function of the LES valve while increasing the number of reflux events. Steroid inhalers may also decrease esophageal resistance to injury.

It is not clear whether gastroesophageal reflux causes asthma on its own, or if asthma medications cause gastroesophageal reflux on their own. It is clear, however, that a vicious cycle exists between asthma and reflux. Reflux causes worsened asthma, causing the need for more medications, causing more reflux, and so on.

Recommendations

1. Talk to your physician about changing or optimizing you asthma medication to reduce your risk for worsening reflux.

2. Adhere to the anti-reflux precautions listed in this manual including raising the head of your bed. Asthmatics are particularly susceptible to the effects of night time reflux. This is why asthmatics are especially helped by elevating the head of their beds.

3. Talk to your physician about temporarily prescribing an anti-acid medication to your treatment regimen to reduce acid production. This medication and a program of anti-reflux precautions may help reduce asthma symptoms, thereby breaking this cycle.

PREGNANCY

As a developing child grows inside of mom's abdomen over nine months, the mom's stomach is slowly squeezed into a smaller and smaller area of the abdomen. Between 40% and 80% of all pregnant women interviewed report very significant heartburn and discomfort when lying down because of reflux. Most of the women with symptoms are between their first and sixth month of pregnancy, although this may vary from person to person.

In addition to having the baby pushing on the stomach to cause reflux, the high levels of progesterone that mom produces during pregnancy also causes reflux. This progesterone acts directly on the LES valve causing it to squeeze less tightly.

Recommendations

1. Common sense and medical knowledge dictate that pregnant moms should limit or avoid medications during pregnancy. Therefore, the emphasis in improving reflux symptoms is placed on general anti-reflux precautions.

2. Elevate the head of your bed, eat frequent small meals, and sleeping on your right side.

3. Elevation of the head of the bed 3-6 inches may have a dramatic effect on reflux symptoms. It is not likely that this degree of elevation will have any negative effects (such as swelling of the feet or varicose veins). Remember that for 12 or more hours per day you are in a vertical position while walking around. Lying with your head slightly elevated at night will still allow fluid to move from your feet to your heart as it normally should. Speak with your obstetrician regarding management of reflux prior to elevating the head of your bed.

medical problems which lead to reflux symptoms

decreased SALIVATION

People with xerostomia (decreased salivation) have an increased likelihood of symptomatic reflux disease. Saliva is important for washing down and neutralizing acid that is refluxed throughout the day. There are a number of conditions which lead to decreased saliva production:

- Sjogren's Syndrome — Dry eyes, dry mouth, a variety of autoimmune phenomena
- Sicca Syndrome — Dry eyes, dry mouth
- Collagen Vascular Disease — Scleroderma having the most pronounced symptoms of reflux
- Radiation Therapy — Radiation to the head and neck for cancer treatment injures saliva glands
- Cystic Fibrosis
- Acquired Immune Deficiency Syndrome

Recommendations

1. Visit your physician for proper management of your health problem.

2. Ask your physician about the various medications that increase salivation, and reduce reflux symptoms.

3. Observe strict anti-reflux precautions if you have a decrease in the production of saliva. Elevating the head of the bed has been shown to help a number of patients in this group.

4. Besides medications to stimulate saliva production, excellent alternatives include using gums and lozenges, artificial saliva, and carrying a water bottle with you at all times.

5. In many of these cases, esophageal irritation or injury will be present necessitating treatment with acid reducing medication. Talk with your physician.

increased acid PRODUCTION

People with increased levels of acid production by the stomach have reflux events that are damaging to the esophagus. If allowed to continue, the damage can involve the LES valve and eventually make reflux even worse. The following is a list of the various conditions and foods which increase acid production in the stomach.

- Zollinger-Ellison Syndrome — very high acid output requiring medical or surgical treatment.
- Duodenal ulcer disease — Persons with excess acid production may develop a duodenal ulcer (an erosion of the small bowel).
- Alcohol intake — Alcohol has been clearly shown to increase acid production.
- Stressful lifestyle.
- Trauma or Surgery — Trauma and surgery stress the body and increase acid production.
- Tobacco use — All tobacco products directly increase acid production.

Recommendations

1. Acid production in some instances may be high enough to warrant immediate medication therapy by your physician to avoid damage to your esophagus and stomach.

2. All of these factors mentioned above are worthy of consult with your physician. In addition to any therapies or cessation programs offered, you should still observe the standard anti-reflux precautions. Such lifestyle modifications will serve you a lifetime and may allow you to avoid medications in the future.

■ ■ ■

swallowing **DISORDERS**

Some individuals have an esophagus which does not properly propel food into the stomach during a swallow. The following are examples of disorders associated with difficulty swallowing:

- Scleroderma — a disorder of skin and collagen which constricts the esophagus.
- Neurological disorders — i.e. Lou Gehrig's disease, multiple sclerosis, polio, muscular dystrophy, selected nerve injuries.
- Brain injury patients.
- Cancers of the head and neck — patients who have surgery or radiation therapy to the throat and/or voice box can have difficulty swallowing.
- Trauma patients — patients who have injured the muscles and nerves associated with swallowing.
- Alcohol — interferes with proper swallowing especially if taken before bed time. or if taken in excess.

Many of these disorders result in poor handling of refluxed stomach acid. The acid is not swallowed or neutralized quickly, as it would be in a person without the particular swallowing problem. This results in prolonged exposure of esophagus to acids.

Recommendations

1. Observe standard anti-reflux precautions, including elevating the head of your bed.

2. Talk to your physician about any current therapies, including physical therapy or speech therapy, which may be available for these problems. If you are experiencing irritation or injury to your esophagus, your physician will prescribe medication to stop the damage and promote healing. Again … it is important to follow the lifestyle guidelines during this phase of treatment as they will serve as a life-long foundation for your therapy.

conditions in which **THE STOMACH EMPTIES** *more slowly than normal*

Fatty meals have been shown to delay emptying of the stomach. Other more uncommon reasons for delayed emptying of the stomach may include diabetes mellitus, stomach ulcer, or a growth within the stomach. These conditions are rarely the main cause of reflux disease, but cases have been reported. Your physician should be recommending diagnostic procedures and treatment for you if he suspects these conditions.

Recommendations

1. Enlist the help of your physician in managing any concurrent health problems and ask if any of these may be leading to slowed emptying of the stomach or worsened reflux.

2. Observe strict anti-reflux precautions. Include elevating the head of your bed only if your physician feels that this position will not negatively influence any of your other health issues.

Burning Fact

Your stomach intestines are about 23 feet in length. The lining of these "digestive tubes" are folded many times to create a large surface on which to digest food. The surface area of the entire digestive track is over 400 square yards, the area of major league baseball infield.

medications **THAT CAN WORSEN** *reflux*

Many physicians and patients are not fully aware that many commonly prescribed medications can worsen and even cause reflux disease. If you are currently taking one or more of the following medications and you have symptomatic reflux, you should speak with your physician about the possibility of an alternative medication or different dosing schedule.

Asthma Medication

- Theophylline
- Bronchodilators (i.e. albuterol)
- Inhaled Corticosteroids
- Ipratropamine bromide inhalers

Anti-Hypertensive Medication

- The nitrate family
- Calcium channel blockers

Sedatives

- Diazepam
- Many other related sedatives

Progesterone

- Found in oral contraceptives
- Elevated in pregnancy

Narcotics

- Meperidine
- Morphine

Tobacco and coffee

- Nicotine
- Caffeine

Recommendations

1. Speak with your physician before stopping or changing any of your medications. Ask your physician if any of your current medications worsen reflux symptoms, and if so, inquire whether alternatives are available.

2. Observe the standard anti-reflux preventions, including elevating the head of your bed.

general daily guidelines to **ALLEVIATE YOUR SYMPTOMS** *of reflux*

This manual has just reviewed the many factors in an individual's lifestyle which may either be causing or contributing to gastroesophageal reflux disease. After each lifestyle factor was discussed, a number of recommendations were offered to improve the likelihood of feeling better.

Here is a helpful summary of the lifestyle recommendations: Check each step as it's incorporated into your lifestyle.

1. Limit or avoid the reflux-producing foods:
- Caffeine
- Fatty foods
- Carbonated Beverages
- Spearmint
- Chocolate
- Alcohol
- Peppermint

2. Decrease the size of each meal. Five to six small meals each day are ideal.

3. Avoid the "Reflux Zone."
- No eating after 7 p.m. You need 3-4 hours of digestion time before retiring to bed.

4. Elevate the head of your bed by 3-6 inches.

5. Tobacco — As discussed previously, tobacco products injure the esophagus and increase reflux. Nicotine gum and patches may also contribute to worsened reflux. Enroll in a smoking cessation program and talk to your physician for help today.

6. Alcohol — Clearly shown in the medical literature to worsen or cause reflux, especially if taken before bed.

7. Stress reduction program
- Daily walks
- Meditation
- Quiet reading
- Soft music
- Take just twenty minutes each day from your 1990's lifestyle to "chill out."

8. Talk to your physician about any of the medications that you are taking that may worsen reflux. We do not recommend changing your medication or dose without speaking to your physician first.

9. Avoid tight clothing around your midsection.

10. Avoid belching, straining, squatting, and bending as much as possible if you already have reflux symptoms.

11. Begin a healthy living and healthy well-being program today!
- Exercise
- Reduce fat intake
- Stop smoking
- Lose weight

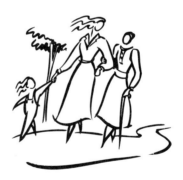

Burning Fact

There are 1.7 million physicians in China - 1 for every 47,640 people. Compare this to Italy where there is 1 physician for every 225 people.

medical *TREATMENT BY YOUR physician*

People are seen by their physicians for symptoms of gastroesophageal reflux routinely. The severity of the problem is assessed by evaluating the symptoms and their duration. Physical examination may include looking at the throat and voice box, looking at the esophagus with a special camera, and possibly looking at the stomach with the same camera. These examinations detect areas of damage from the reflux. A special test is sometimes ordered to detect acid in the throat and esophagus. It is called a pH probe study. Occasionally, an x-ray examination called a barium esophogram is required.

There are four general phases that physicians use to treat patients with reflux. These phases should be thought of as stair steps in treatment. Most patients start out with step one or Phase One and may have satisfactory relief of their symptoms. Others require further treatment in Phases Two, Three, and Four.

The following is a brief explanation of each phase:

Phase One
Lifestyle management and reflux precautions with occasional liquid antacid use.

Phase Two
Addition of medications called H-2 Blockers (block acid production) and more liberal use of antacid preparations.

Phase Three
Addition of stronger acid-blocking agents like omeprazole and other medications which increase the speed of stomach emptying.

Phase Four
Surgery to correct gastroesophageal reflux disease.

We will now review each of these phases of treatment and look at the costs to you, the medical consumer, associated with each phase.

treatment **PHASES**
FOR *gastroesophageal reflux*

Phase One

This phase relies entirely on general anti-reflux precautions to reduce reflux symptoms. After having read this manual, you are now an expert on anti-reflux precautions. These precautions include such things as avoiding late-night eating and elevating the head of your bed. This phase is the basis for all patients with reflux. Phase one therapy may also include the occasional use of over-the-counter antacid preparation during periods of heartburn symptoms. These precautions should be employed by all patients with reflux before any perscription medications are begun and should be continued during any medicl or surgical therapies.

Quotes from the medical literature:

During the last few years, we have seen the advent of new technologies in the diagnosis and treatment of gastroesophageal reflux disease. A better understanding of the pathophysiological nature of the disease has afforded a number of new therapeutic options, particularly potent and effective acid suppressing medications. With these alternatives, less emphasis is now placed on simplistic traditional modes of therapy, such as diet modification, antacid use, postural measures, and drug restriction. Perhaps this tendency to disregard the older, more conservative therapies is a mistake. *Kitchen, Castell. Archives of Internal Medicine 1991;151:448-454.* (reprinted with permission)

Therapy should be instituted by recommending several changes in lifestyle ... many patients find that these changes reduce or eliminate the symptoms of reflux. Elevation of the head of the bed has been found to result in subjective and objective improvement in reflux; the degree of improvement approaches that associated with therapy with histamine receptor blockers (i.e, ranitidine). *Pope CE. The New England Journal of Medicine. 1994; 331 (10): 656-660.* (reprinted with permission)

Most individuals (as high as 90%) will experience complete relief of their symptoms if they adhere to anti-reflux precautions. There are, of course, some patients who require the next steps in therapy if Phase One alone is not sufficient. Some patients may also have damage to their esophagus when they first come to the attention of a physician. These persons require Phase Two or Phase Three treatment right away. Your physician will make this determination.

Remember, lifestyle management is the basis for treating reflux, even if you need short-term medication treatment. Such non-pharmacological and inexpensive strategies will give you a lifetime of disease prevention and may lessen your need for medications.

treatment **PHASES**
FOR *gastroesophageal reflux*

Phase Two

H-2 Blockers include the medications ranitidine (Zantac®), cimetidine (Tagamet®), famotidine (Pepcid®), and nizatidine (Axid®). These drugs block one of the ways in which the stomach is stimulated to produce acid. They are used to treat reflux induced esophageal irritation, gastritis, stomach ulcers, and duodenal ulcers. They are some of the most commonly prescribed medications in the world.

The medical literature states that the dose of H-2 blocker needed to treat esophageal injury is frequently many times higher than that needed to treat other problems, such as gastritis or peptic ulcer disease. Ask your physician if your dosage regimen is the right one for your problem.

Physicians will occasionally start reflux patients on both anti-reflux precautions (Phase One) and H-2 Blockers (Phase Two) at the time of their <u>first</u> visit. This would seem warranted as long as the patient has evidence of esophageal injury or such severe symptoms that it would be unwise to wait before starting medication. The medical literature supports that it is safe for most patients to have a 2-3 month trial of Phase One anti-reflux treatment prior to any drug therapy, as long as symptoms or tests do not reveal severe disease or esophageal injury.

Over-the-counter antacid preparations are also a common therapy in reflux treatment. Some physicians include antacids in phase one of treatment to be used only when symptoms arise. In phase two, antacids are used more regularly, usually 1-2 tablespoons one hour after meals and again before bed-time. Unfortunately, antacids have not been universally shown to reduce reflux damage or to promote healing, but many people report that the antacids alleviate their symptoms. Remember, antacids are medications with potential side effects (see page 69). Ask your physician about any possible interactions with your current medications.

A recent study published in the *New England Journal of Medicine* found that patients who first present with severe symptoms and already have signs of esophagus injury should be treated early with phase three medications (see page 67).

treatment **PHASES**
FOR *gastroesophageal reflux*

Phase Three

If Phases One and Two have not provided satisfactory relief or have not allowed healing to begin in the esophagus, the next phase utilizes medications which totally block acid production in the stomach. The medications are called omeprazole (Prilosec®) and lansoprazole (Prevacid®). These medications are more modern than the traditional H-2 Blockers. It has been shown to promote healing even more quickly and effectively than H-2 Blockers.

The use of omeprazole was originally limited to six weeks or less because of a remote likelihood of developing a certain type of growth noted in the animals which it was initially tested. Many gastroenterologists and other experts in the field, however, are continuing this medication for longer then six weeks. They are appropriately basing the decision on the fact that the likelihood of such a growth is infinitely rare, and that many patients will suffer complications from reflux without the medication. Recent investigations are further supporting the use of omeprazole for periods up to one year or longer.

Motility agents are medications that speed up the emptying of the stomach and possibly increase the function of the LES valve. These include metoclopramide (Reglan®) and cisapride. These drugs have been shown to reduce reflux signs and symptoms, usually when added to a regimen of acid-blocking medications like omeprazole (Prilosec®).

treatment **PHASES**
FOR *gastroesophageal reflux*

Phase Four

There is a group of people who simply can not relieve their reflux symptoms or stop the continuing damage to their esophagus despite all the efforts of Phases One, Two and Three. For these individuals, surgery is the final and often most successful option. There are a number of surgical procedures which either tighten the LES valve or alter the nerve supply to the stomach to reduce acid production. General surgeons perform this procedure and are the experts at managing reflux cases which simply will not improve with lifestyle changes or medication.

Many surgeons are now performing surgery for intractable reflux via a laparoscope technique (a tiny telescope inserted into the abdomen). This procedure is in its early stages, but will undoubtedly serve to reduce post-operative discomfort, hospitalization time, and costs.

General surgeons and gastroenterologists are beginning to recommend anti-reflux surgery earlier and more frequently because minimally invasive, laparoscopic techniques have shown success and are better accepted by patients. Long-term use of medication is reduced in most patients who have this surgery.

Surgery for reflux is often successful. Patients may experience relief of symptoms for as long as five to ten years. Many of these patients require either fewer medications or no further medications after reflux surgery. Surgery is not without risk and is generally reserved only for the person with intractable reflux who show evidence of esophageal injury.

H-2 blockers / *ANTACIDS*

Be aware of the following when taking H-2 Blockers or Antacids:

H-2 Blockers

1. There are possible interactions of some H-2 blockers (cimetidine) with the body's ability to metabolize other drugs. Tell your physician if you are currently taking H-2 blockers with any other medication including: Warfarin, Benzodiazepines, Lidocaine, Metronidazole, Phenytoin, Triamterene, Tricyclic Antidepressants, and Theophylline.

2. The cost of H-2 blockers can be quite high, especially since dosage recommendations for reflux are usually 2-4 times the usual dose. Some agents are as costly as $2,800 per year.

3. Antacid use may affect absorption of H-2 blockers.

4. Short-term treatment. Most H-2 blockers are not recommended for periods longer than eight weeks. Most patients, however, require longer periods of therapy.

Antacids

1. The stomach may increase acid production **above normal** one to two hours after taking some antacid preparations.

2. Calcium-containing antacids may cause higher than normal calcium levels, especially in the patient with kidney disease.

3. Magnesium-containing antacids have a laxative effect which can cause diarrhea.

4. Aluminum-containing antacids are constipating, which can cause impaction or obstruction in certain higher risk patients.

5. Sodium bicarbonate antacids can cause flatulence (gas) and stomach fullness.

6. A one-year supply of antacid can be costly, as much as $1,000.

7. Antacids may alter the effects of certain drugs including H-2 blockers, Digoxin, Indomethecin, Iron, Tetracycline, and Naprosyn.

8. High-sodium contents in some antacids may cause problems in patients with heart, kidney or blood pressure problems.

cost comparison of the *PHASES OF TREATMENT* for reflux

Phase One
- Reflux precautions are simple, conservative therapies and are virtually cost free.
- Reflux precautions are a life-long treatment, unlike some of the drug and surgical treatments.

Phase Two
- H-2 Blockers are taken between one and three times per day
- The dosages used in the following cost estimate are a range from the normal dose for ulcer disease to the higher dose for reflux induced esophageal injury

	Ranitidine	Nizatidine	Famotidine	Cimetidine
Cost per month	$ 80-240	$ 60-120	$ 80-240	$ 80-160
Cost per year	$ 960-2880	$ 720-1440	$ 960-2880	$960-1920

- Antacids taken as directed for reflux are about $80 per month and $960 per year

Phase Three
- Omeprazole is taken once per day, either 20 mg. or 40 mg. per day.

Cost per month	$ 100-200
Cost per year	$ 1200-2400

- Cisapride is taken four times per day

Cost per month	$ 80-100
Cost per year	$ 960-1200

Phase Four

Surgery is the most expensive of the therapies if you consider the one-time cost. Actually, surgery can be very effective in resolving symptoms of reflux and can have lasting effects for 5-10 years. During those symptom-free years many individuals do not require medications. This saving must be considered when analyzing costs.

Surgical costs, including hospitalization (7-10 days) and follow-up, can exceed $40,000.

Many surgeons are now performing surgery for intractable reflux via a laparoscope technique (a tiny telescope inserted into the abdomen). This technique has been deemed "minimally invasive anti-reflux surgery." This procedure is in its early stages, but will undoubtedly serve to reduce post-operative discomfort, hospitalization time, and costs.

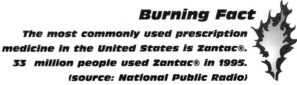

Burning Fact

The most commonly used prescription medicine in the United States is Zantac®. 33 million people used Zantac® in 1995. (source: National Public Radio)

■ ■ ■

nutrition **AND**
gastroesophageal
REFLUX DISEASE

Nutrition plays a predominant role in managing the symptoms of GERD. Certain foods directly cause reflux events or can mimic reflux symptoms. Being overweight can make an individual more likely to have GERD.

This section will review the topic of weight loss and provide examples of reflux inducing and reducing menus. You will then find recipes of low-fat, low-reflux foods that we are sure you'll enjoy.

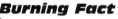

Burning Fact

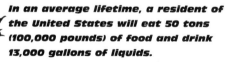

In an average lifetime, a resident of the United States will eat 50 tons (100,000 pounds) of food and drink 13,000 gallons of liquids.

HOW DO I *lose weight?*

It seems that this is America's burning question. We are flooded with television commercials for exercise equipment, diet centers, weight-loss milkshakes, and fat-free foods. We are told by our physicians that it is imperative to be at one's ideal body weight in order to avoid many of the diseases of an affluent society, namely heart disease, cancer, and diabetes.

Most people have tried some form of exercise or diet plan to shed a few pounds. The result, unfortunately, is usually temporary weight loss followed by regaining the lost pounds (and often a few extra).

This book is designed to inform you about gastroesophageal reflux disease and to give you the most up-to-date information to help minimize your heartburn symptoms. Being overweight is a known cause of heartburn (see page xx). Eating high-fat foods also leads to worsened heartburn (see page xx). Here is an introduction to some of the basic facts you should know to make your weight loss and fitness programs successful.

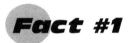

Fact #1

A calorie is a measure of energy.

You can **consume** one calorie by taking in 3 Cherrios ®, a 1/2 teaspoon of soda, 1/10 of a mint, or 1/500 of a burrito.

You can **expend** one calorie by walking briskly for 10 seconds, climbing 6 steps, or sweeping the floor for 6 seconds.

Your average daily calorie requirement depends on your weight, sex, body type and activity level. Most women need about 2000 calories per day. Men need about 2500 calories per day.

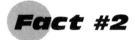

Fact #2

When you consume (eat) more than you expend (burn), your body stores the extra energy as fat.

The food you eat is like the gasoline you put in your car's tank. Your car, however, can only store a certain amount of gasoline. Imagine, for a moment, that your car has a new feature. Your car now has extra expandable gas tanks in the trunk (your rear end), fenders (your saddle bags), and doors (your love handles). As you over-fill your gas tank, these expandable tanks swell to hold any amount of extra gas (energy).

If you drive the car 20 miles in one day, you usually put in enough gas to fill the tank, say one gallon. But let's say that every day you put in one and a half gallons, still driving only 20 miles per day. That means that every day you'll have an extra 1/2 gallon of gas (energy) stored in the extra tanks (fat).

Now at first, the expandable tanks will not dramatically alter the appearance of your car. It will remain a sleek, svelte machine. But how about after six months of storing that extra 1/2 gallon per day? By then your saddle bags are hanging, you can't close your trunk, and your love handles require two hands!

Your car now weighs 80 gallons or 560 pounds more than it did before you started over-filling it and under-running it! The same thing can happen to you when you start over-eating and under-exercising.

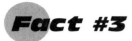

Fact #3

Eating an excess 3500 calories is needed to store one pound of body fat,

How much food is 3500 calories? How about:
- 12 slices of cheese pizza or
- 24 sodas (an entire case) or
- 2 bags of tortilla chips or
- 29 glasses of 2% milk or
- 25 glasses of sweetened iced tea.

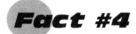

Fact #4

The concept of weight loss can be simplified by taking small, easy steps every day toward reducing your intake and increasing your activity.

Eat 100 calories more than you burn every day for a year and you can expect to be carrying around an **extra** 10 pounds by the new year.

Remove 100 calories from your meal plan every day for a year and you'll be walking with a step that's 10 pounds **lighter** by year's end!

Walk just 30 minutes every day for a year and you can expect to be walking 15 pounds lighter on your feet by the new year.

Let's put this into perspective. Imagine that you have a regular 12 ounce soda with your lunch every day for one year. That's 150 calories per day just from the soda. Most sodas are at least twice that large (300 calories), but we'll give you the benefit of the doubt and say yours was a "small" and you didn't have three free refills. Drinking that daily soda will add up to a quite a few extra pounds by year's end. How many? About 15 pounds! Your body sees this excess food as extra gasoline that isn't burned by the body's engine, so the energy is stored as fat. Where does it get stored? You guessed it...right in your saddle bags, your rear end, and your love handles.

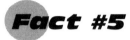

Fact #5

Physical activity of any type has the effect of regulating appetite.

A common argument heard from individuals who are reluctant to start an exercise program is, "Why should I walk every day? I'll only burn calories during the walk itself. I'll be so hungry afterwards that I'll eat twice as much."

If you engage in any type of physical activity, a number of things happen. First, activity of any type will suppress appetite. Activity will alleviate boredom, tension, and anxiety, all of which can lead to overeating. Physical activity will occupy a small segment of your time each day, making it unlikely that you'll be eating or watching television during those exercise periods.

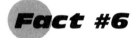

Fact #6

Daily physical activity will increase your overall metabolism.

When you exercise, your body needs to increase its ability to transport nutrients to the muscular system, as well as its ability to utilize (burn) those calories. Your body will also increase the amount of muscle tissue to allow it to perform these daily physical activities more efficiently. This combination of events will allow your body to burn more calories 24 hours a day, in addition to the time when you're exercising. This further promotes weight loss and fitness.

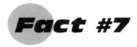 Fact #7

Keep it simple.

The biggest mistake most people make in approaching fitness and weight loss is that of making the process more complicated than it is.

You really don't need the latest diet book, the latest aerobics video, or the latest nutritional supplement. Most importantly, don't feel that you need to spend a dime to lose weight. The only added expense is a good pair of shoes in which to walk a mile a day.

Remember the simple facts mentioned above. If you eat more than you burn, you'll be adding to your saddle bags. Burn more than you eat, and you'll likely to be stepping lighter by year's end. How much more simple could it be than taking the following steps:

1. Sind something in your regular meals and habits that's worth about 150 calories and simply eliminate it from your plan. Any food that you don't require for essential nutrients will do such as your daily soda or potato chips.

2. Make the time in your day to do something active that you don't currently do on a regular basis. The activity that you choose should burn 150 calories or more. Examples are walking one mile at 4.5 mph, walking 1.5 miles at 2 mph, gardening for 45 minutes, or swimming for 30 minutes. (See section on activities and the calories burned page 79).

Either of these steps will take 10-15 pounds out of your saddle bags by the new year. Taken together you may find double that weight loss!

Always check with your physician before beginning any weight loss or exercise plan.

Burning Fact

The Hawaiian Ironman™ is an endurance triathlon event consisting of a 2.4-mile ocean swim, a 112-mile bike race, and a 26.2-mile marathon run. Competitors take 8-17 hours to complete this event and can burn as many as 1500 Kcal/hour. The total calories expended in this event would be the equivalent of 4 cases of cola, 8 large pizzas, or 200 bananas.

how many *CALORIES* can i burn in *THIRTY* minutes?

Activity	Calories Burned
Sleeping	*36*
Watching Television	*36*
Standing	*42*
General Housework	*123*
Washing Windows	*126*
Mopping Floor	*138*
Light Gardening	*108*
Mowing Lawn (power)	*123*
Mowing Lawn (manual)	*135*
Shoveling Snow	*234*
Walking 2 mph	*105*
Walking 4.5 mph	*201*
Walking upstairs	*525*
Running 7 mph	*423*
Bicycling 5.5 mph	*150*
Bicycling 13 mph	*321*
Dancing (moderate)	*126*
Dancing (vigorous)	*171*
Skiing (cross-country)	*351*
Swimming 20 yd/min.	*144*
Tennis	*201*

These values are estimates of caloric expenditure per 30 minutes for a 150 pound person. If you weigh more than 150 pounds, your expenditure may be slightly more. If you weigh less, your expenditure may be slightly less.

■ ■ ■

---

samples of meals

LIKELY *to* PROMOTE
reflux symptoms

BREAKFAST
Fried Eggs
Biscuit with Jam and Butter
Bacon
Whole Milk
Coffee (regular or decaffeinated)

LUNCH
Grilled Ham and Cheese Sandwich
Potato Chips
Chocolate Brownie
Cola (regular or decaffeinated)

SNACKS
Nacho Chips
Doughnuts
Candy Bars
Cheese and Crackers
Croissant
Bagel with Cream Cheese (regular)

DINNER
Grilled Steak
French Fries
Garden Salad with Ranch Dressing
Red Wine

Dessert
Chocolate Cheese Cake
Chocolate Chip Cookies
Ice Cream
Chocolate Candy
Pecan Pie

samples of meals
LIKELY *to* PREVENT
reflux symptoms

BREAKFAST
Vegetable Omelet (egg whites only)
Cereal with non-fat Milk
Toast with Jam
Banana
Non-fat Milk
Herbal Tea (no caffeine)

LUNCH
Turkey Sandwich
  (mustard, tomato, sprouts)
Pretzels
Yogurt (low fat)
Grapes
Non-fat Milk

SNACKS
Pretzels / Popcorn (air popped)
Yogurt (low fat)
Raisins
Low-fat Granola Bars
Low-fat Fruit and Grain Bars
Low-fat Cookies (fig, molasses, ginger)
Any Fresh Fruit

DINNER
Grilled Barbecue Chicken Breast
Baked Potato with non-fat Sour Cream
Garden Salad with non-fat Dressing
Baked Apple
Fruit Juice or Decaffeinated Iced Tea

■ ■ ■

LOW-FAT *recipes* *designed to* AVOID REFLUX *producing foods*

French Toast

    4 egg whites, beaten
    1/4 cup skim milk
    1/4 tsp. vanilla extract
    6 slices of bread
    cinnamon

Mix egg whites, milk, and vanilla extract. Soak bread in mixture for 2-3 minutes. Brown bread slices on a griddle or Teflon pan (spray with non-stick cooking spray if necessary). Sprinkle each serving with cinnamon, and serve with syrup, powdered sugar, honey, or jam.

Orange Streusel Coffee Cake

    2 cups sifted flour
    1/2 cup sugar
    2 tsp. baking powder
    1 1/2 Tbsp. grated orange rind
    2 egg whites, beaten
    1/2 cup skim milk
    1/2 cup orange juice
    1/3 cup vegetable oil

Mix flour, sugar, baking powder, and orange rind. Set aside. In a separate bowl, mix the remaining ingredients. Gradually stir the wet ingredients into the dry until the mixture is dampened, but still somewhat lumpy. Spray 8 x 8 x 2 inch cake pan with non-stick cooking spray. Pour batter into pan.

low-fat, low-reflux
RECIPES

Streusel Topping

1/4 cup flour
1/2 cup sugar or brown sugar
2 Tbsp. low calorie margarine

Mix flour and sugar together. Cut in margarine. Sprinkle topping over batter and bake at 375" for 30 to 40 minutes (when browned).

Fresh Chicken Salad

2 cups cooked chicken, diced
1/2 cup celery, diced
1/4 cup green pepper, diced
3 scallions, sliced
1/4 cup pimiento, chopped
1/2 cucumber, peeled and diced
1 small tomato, diced
1/4 cup non-fat mayonnaise
1 Tbsp. lemon juice
salt and pepper
paprika

Mix vegetables, chicken, mayonnaise, lemon juice, salt and pepper to taste. Serve on a bed of fresh salad greens and garnish with paprika, or on a whole wheat sandwich roll for a delicious lunch.

■ ■ ■

low-fat, low-reflux
RECIPES

Beef, Barley, and Vegetable Soup
    3/4 pound lean beef (trim and cut into cubes)
    2 (14 1/2 oz) cans beef broth
    2 Tbsp. herbed vinegar
    1 tsp. dried tarragon
    1 tsp. salt
    1/4 tsp. pepper
    3/4 cup quick cooking barley
    1 (10 oz) package frozen mixed vegetables

In a large pot, add steak to 4 cups of cold water. Bring to a boil. Skim off any fat that accumulates on the surface. Add broth, vinegar, and seasonings. Cover and simmer for one hour Add barley, cover and cook 25 min.Add vegetables, cover and cook until they are tender, about 5 to 10 min.

Stuffed Shells
    12 ounces large pasta shells
    2 Tbsp. olive oil
    1/4 lb. fresh mushrooms, chopped
    2 egg whites
    1/2 lb. non-fat Ricotta Cheese (or non-fat cottage cheese, blended)
    3/4 cup part-skim mozzarella cheese, shredded
    1 tsp. dried basil
    1/2 tsp. salt
    1/4 tsp. pepper
    3 cups marinara sauce

Cook shells in a large pot of boiling water until tender, but still firm. Drain and rinse under cold water. In a large skillet or wok, heat oil over med-high heat. Add mushrooms and saute for 3 to 4 minutes. Remove to a bowl.In a separate mixing bowl, mix egg whites, cheeses, and seasonings. Add mushrooms and mix. Pour marinara sauce into skillet and heat over medium setting. Fill shells with cheese mixture and place over sauce.Reduce heat to low. Cover and cook for 30 minutes.

low-fat, low-reflux
RECIPES

Sunday Chicken Dinner

4 chicken breasts
4 medium-size potatoes, peeled and sliced 1/2 inches thick
2 large carrots, peeled and quartered lengthwise
1/2 lb. fresh green beans, cut into 2 inch pieces
1 large onion, diced
1 clove garlic, crushed
1 Tbsp. dried parsley flakes
salt and pepper
1/2 cup cooking sherry

In a large oven-ware pot, layer ingredients in this order: chicken, potato slices, carrots, garlic, onions, and green beans. Sprinkle with parsley, salt & pepper. Pour sherry over all ingredients and cover. Bake at 300° F for 2 to 2 1/2 hours, until vegetables are tender.(The alcohol in the sherry will evaporate during cooking, leaving only the flavor & tenderizing properties which enhance this dish.)

Oatmeal Raisin Cookies

1 cup flour, sifted
1/2 tsp. baking soda
1 1/2 cups quick cooking oats
2 egg whites, beaten slightly
1/2 teaspoon cinnamon
1 cup brown sugar
1/3 cup vegetable oil
1/2 cup skim milk
1 tsp. vanilla extract
1 cup raisins

Mix together flour, baking soda, and oats in a large mixing bowl. In a separate bowl, combine egg whites, cinnamon, sugar, oil, milk, vanilla, and raisins. Gradually mix wet ingredients with the dry ingredients. Spray cookie sheet with non-stick cooking spray. Drop teaspoon sized portions of the batter onto the cookie sheet. Bake at 375° for 12 to 15 minutes. (Shorter cooking time will make chewier cookies).

■ ■ ■

low-fat, low-reflux
RECIPES

Honey-Baked Apples
    4 Granny Smith apples
    1/4 cup honey
    1/4 cup orange or lemon juice
    1/4 cup water
    1 tsp. grated lemon or orange rind (optional)

Wash and core apples, and place in an ovenproof dish. Combine remaining ingredients and pour over apples. Bake apples at 375°, covered for for one half hour. Baste as needed.

Fresh Fruit Cup
    4 cups sliced fresh fruit (apples, bananas,
    berries, grapefruit, grapes, oranges,
    pears, and melons)
    3 Tbsp. frozen orange juice concentrate
    Grapenuts® cereal

Prepare fruit, then mix with the orange juice. Chill for one to two hours. Sprinkle with Grapenuts® prior to serving.

low-fat, low-reflux

RECIPES

Hearty Chicken Vegetable Soup

3 Tbsp. olive oil

1 pound skinless, boneless chicken breasts

(trim any fat and cut into 1-inch cubes)

1 medium onion, chopped

1 garlic clove, minced

1 carrot, sliced

1 medium zucchini, diced

3 cans low-fat chicken broth

1 (14 1/2 ounce) can crushed tomatoes

1 tsp. salt

1 tsp. dried basal

1/2 cup long-grain white rice

1 cup frozen corn

In a large pot, heat 1 1/2 Tbsp. of the olive oil over medium-high heat. Add chicken and cook, stirring, until meat is white but still moist, 3 to 5 minutes. Remove to a plate. In the same pot, add the remaining 1 1/2 Tbsp. of olive oil and heat, swirling oil to coat bottom of pan. Add onion, garlic, carrot, and zucchini, stirring until softened, 3 to 5 minutes.

Add chicken broth, crushed tomatoes, salt, basil, and 1 1/2 cups water. Cook on medium-high for 2 minutes and then reduce heat to medium-low. Add rice, cover, and cook for 40 minutes.

Add chicken and corn. Stir and let simmer 5 minutes or until rice is tender and chicken is hot.

■ ■ ■

low-fat, low-reflux

RECIPES

Halibut in an Orange Sauce

1 pound halibut steak, cut 1/2 - 3/4 inch thick
1/2 cup onion, chopped
1 clove garlic, minced
1 Tbsp. margarine
2 Tbsp fresh parsley, chopped
3/4 tsp. orange rind
1/4 tsp. salt
1/8 tsp. pepper
1/4 cup orange juice

Preheat oven to 400. Arrange fish in a single layer in an 8x8x2 inch baking dish, set aside. Saute onion and garlic in margarine until tender, 3 to 4 minutes. Remove from heat and stir in parsley, orange rind, salt and pepper. Spread this mixture over fish. Sprinkle orange juice over all. Cover and bake for 15 to 20 minutes or until fish flakes easily with a fork.

Rosemary Baked Chicken

4 skinless, boneless chicken breast halves (approx. 4 ounces each)
1 cup low-fat saltine cracker crumbs
1/4 tsp salt
1/8 tsp pepper
1/2 tsp rosemary
2 egg whites
2 Tbsp cold water

Preheat oven to 400. In shallow pan, combine cracker crumbs, salt, pepper, and rosemary. Set aside. In a shallow bowl, beat egg whites with water. Dip chicken in egg white mixture and then roll in seasoned crumbs. Spray baking dish with a non-stick spray. Place chicken in baking dish. Pieces should not touch. Bake for 40 to 50 minutes or until chicken is cooked through and tender.

low-fat, low-reflux
RECIPES

Foil Baked Fish Fillets

4 Fillets (approx 2 lbs.)
1 Tbsp. Margarine or vegetable oil
1/4 cup green onions, chopped
1/2 pound fresh mushrooms, sliced
2 Tbsp. lemon juice
1 Tbsp. fresh dill, chopped
1 Tbsp. parsley, chopped
salt/ pepper

Preheat oven to 400. Saute green onions in margarine until soft (2 to 3 minutes). Add mushrooms and cook an additional 3 to 5 minutes. Stir in lemon juice, dill and parsley, cooking until most of liquid evaporates. Spray 4 pieces of aluminum foil with a non-stick cooking spray. Place a fillet on each piece of foil, season with salt and pepper as desired.

Spoon equal amount of mushroom sauce over each fillet. Seal each piece of foil around the fillets. Bake fillets for 15 to 20 minutes or until fish flakes easily with a fork. Remove to a hot platter and garnish with parsley sprigs and lemon wedges.

glossary of **TERMS**

Asthma: A disorder affecting adults and children in which the small airways of the lungs are reactive to environmental or unknown stimuli which cause the airways to constrict or tighten. This tightening of the airways makes breathing extremely difficult. Asthma patients have a very high likelihood of having significant reflux which can lead to worsening of their asthma symptoms.

Barrett's Esophagus: The cells that line the esophagus are sensitive to the acid from the stomach and may change their shape and function when exposed to repeated episodes of acid reflux. These changes are called metaplasia, some of which are pre-cancerous changes.

Dysphagia: Difficulty swallowing; usually secondary either to stricture of the esophagus, a foreign body, cancer, nerve disorder, or injury to the esophagus.

Edema: Swelling from irritation or inflammation.

Enzymes: Proteins produced in the stomach, liver and pancreas which are released into the digestive tract. These enzymes break down the components of the food we eat.

Erosion: Thinning of the lining of the esophagus from constant reflux exposure to acid and enzymes. Can result in ullceration and bleeding

Erythema: Redness from irritation or inflammation.

Esophageal Dysmotility: Difficulty swallowing secondary to poor coordination of the esophagus muscles.

Esophagitis: Irritation of the esophagus lining, caused frequently by reflux. Can lead to pre-cancerous changes in the esophagus or to bleeding of the esophagus.

Esophagus: The swallowing tube which connects the throat to the stomach. Can become irritated and eroded with repeated reflux.

Gastritis: Irritation of the stomach usually caused by a decrease in the protective layer which covers the inside of the stomach. Can be caused by cigarette smoking, alcohol use, stress, medications, or infections. Can lead to ulcer disease.

Gastroenterologist: Physician who has completed a medical residency and a gastroenterology fellowship. These specialists manage disorders of the gastrointestinal system (digestion disorders.)

Gastroesophageal Reflux Disease: The process of reverse flow of stomach contents (acids and enzymes) into the esophagus thereby causing a variety of symptoms and possible long term injury to the esophagus and other structures.

Gerontologist (Geriatric Medicine): A physician who diagnoses and manages illnesses in the elderly population.

GERD: Gastroesophageal Reflux Disease

Globus Sensation: Sensation of a foreign body or irritation in the throat or voice box, when on examination there is no evidence of such a process.

Heartburn: The sensation of burning in the chest or throat, fullness, "gas bloating," indigestion, pressure in the chest. This is the most common symptom of gastroesophageal reflux, but is also a common symptom of heart disease and impending heart attack. For any symptoms of reflux that persist, including heartburn, you should see your physician to be sure that you do not have another reason to be having this discomfort.

Larynx: Voice Box. You can feel your voice box by placing your finger on your "Adam's apple." This is the top of the voice box.

Lower Esophageal Sphincter: Referred to as the LES valve in this manual. The LES valve is the muscular area at the junction of the esophagus and the stomach. It serves to limit flow of stomach contents back into the esophagus.

Odynophagia: Painful swallowing; usually secondary either to stricture of the esophagus, injury to the esophagus from reflux, irritation or infection of the throat or esophagus, esophageal spasm, cancer in the upper breathing or swallowing tract, foreign body, or spasm of the LES valve.

Otolaryngologist: Physician who has performed a five-to six-year surgical residency specializing in surgery and therapy of disorders of the head and neck. Also Head and Neck surgeon, Ear, Nose and Throat specialist.

Pediatrician: Physician who has completed residency training in diagnosing and managing diseases of young patents, generally patients under the age of eighteen.

pH Probe Study: Minimally invasive test performed by gastroenterologists where a small tube is passed into the esophagus through the nose. This is done to detect acid reflux.

Pulmonologist: Physician who has trained in internal medicine and then completed specialized training in deceases of the respiratory system. They manage such illnesses as asthma, pneumonia, chronic lung disease, cystic fibrosis, etc.

Reflux Precautions: The many non-drug, non-surgical, and cost-free ways in which you can alter your lifestyle to safely and effectively reduce or eliminate reflux disease. See manual for details.

Rheumatologist: Physician who trained in internal medicane and then completed specialized training in inflammatory disease management. They manage such illnesses as arthritis, lupus, scleroderma, etc.

Scleroderma: A collagen vascular disease in which the connective tissues and vessels in the body are inflamed and scarred. Scleroderma affects reflux in that these individuals have a very difficult time swallowing. This problem also makes it difficult to swallow acid that is refluxed into the esophagus from the stomach.

Stomach: The hollow organ which holds swallowed food while digestion begins downstream in the intestines. Food is slowly released as room becomes available in the intestines.

Stricture: Narrowing. A stricture may develop in the esophagus from repeated irritation and burn by reflux. A stricture would make swallowing either difficult or impossible.

Ulcer: Crater-like erosion of the lining of the stomach, esophagus, or duodenum.

APPENDIX 1

Elevating the head of your bed

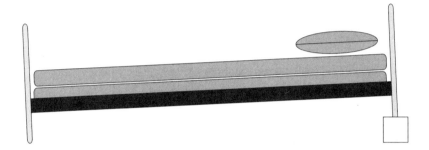

Suggestions: Bricks
Phone Books
Blocks of wood

- Use a stable, wide-based item to raise the head of the bed 4-6 inches.

- Use caution when elevating the bed to avoid back-strain or injury.

- Use caution so that the bed does not become dislodged from the support resulting in injury.

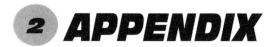

2 *APPENDIX*

Smoking Cessation Groups

American Cancer Society
1599 Clifton Road, N.E.
Atlanta, GA 30329-4251

The American Cancer Society will provide the information necessary for you to meet with smoking cessation groups in your local area. They will also send you free materials on smoking cessation.

National Cancer Institute
9000 Rockville Pike
Building 31, Room 4A-18
Bethesda, MD 20892
1-800-4-CANCER

American Heart Association
National Center
7320 Greenville Avenue
Dallas, TX 75231
(214) 373-6300

Office on Smoking and Health
Centers for Disease Control and Prevention
Mail Stop K-50
4770 Buford Highway NE
(404) 488-5701

American Lung Association
1740 Broadway
New York, NY 10019-4374
(212) 315-8700

APPENDIX 3

Finding your ideal body weight

The following is a chart that you can use to determine your ideal body weight based upon your height and body frame size. Weights are in pounds.

Men

Height	Small Frame	Medium Frame	Large Frame
5'2"	131	136	144
5'3"	133	138	146
5'4"	135	140	149
5'5"	137	142	152
5'6"	139	145	155
5'7"	141	151	158
5'8"	144	154	162
5'9"	146	156	165
5'10"	149	157	169
5'11"	151	160	172
6'0"	155	163	176
6'1"	158	167	180
6'2"	162	171	184
6'3"	165	175	189
6'4"	169	179	194

Women

Height	Small Frame	Medium Frame	Large Frame
4'10"	106	115	125
4'11"	108	117	127
5'0"	109	119	129
5'1"	112	122	132
5'2"	114	125	135
5'3"	117	128	139
5'4"	120	131	142
5'5"	123	134	146
5'6"	126	137	149
5'7"	129	140	153
5'8"	133	143	156
5'9"	135	146	159
5'10"	138	149	162
5'11"	141	152	165
6'0"	144	155	168

This is a compilation of multiple charts used to estimate ideal body weight. Such charts are developed by insurance companies and are based upon the ideal weights which have been shown to minimize disease and mortality.

Ordering:

please contact:
Stop the Heartburn
PO BOX 620891
Woodside CA, 94062

cost:
$9.95 each
$2.00 shipping and handling

checks payable to:
Lagado Publishing

please call:
Stop the Heartburn
415.562.3800

please fax:
Stop the Heartburn
415.562.3800

PLEASE SEND

_____ copies of **Stop the Heartburn** @ $9.95 each to:

Your Name: _____

Address: _____

City: _____ State: _____ Zip: _____

Check ☐   Master Card ☐   Money Order ☐   Visa ☐

Card Number ☐☐☐☐ ☐☐☐☐ ☐☐☐☐ ☐☐☐☐

Cardholder Signature: _____   ☐☐–☐☐

Please make sure that we are shipping to a street address. We cannot ship to a P.O. Box.   Expiration Date

Send this order form with check, money order or card number to:

Stop the Heartburn
Lagado Publishing
P.O. Box 620891 Woodside, CA 94062

Amount _____ copies x $9.95 = _____

Californians add 8.25% sales tax = _____

_____ copies x $2.00 shipping and handling = _____

U.S. funds only, please   TOTAL = _____